Simple Changes for Your Healthy Mind and Relationships

By LaTonya Neely, CSN, CDCES

ISBN- 978-0-9975042-6-2

Library of Congress Control Number 2021908021

Printed and bound in the United States of America

First Printing May 2020

Editing, book cover design and interior formatting by:
Dean Diaries Publishing

To order additional copies of this book, contact the author:

Wellness Choice LLC
mygreenleaf4@gmail.com
www.yellpower.org

Table of Contents

DEDICATION

To my LORD and Savior, Jesus Christ, my patient husband, and our supportive and understanding sons.

Thank you, Dr. Tony Evans, my Texas family with OCBF team and Pastor Greg Bruce, the best church in Missouri, for awesome teaching and prayers.

Introduction

Conflicting Communication in the Church

As a PK (Preacher's kid), I have seen, heard, and felt the goodness of God. I have seen people sharing the good word about how God has brought them out of the darkness and witnessed others giving their lives to Christ. That is a beautiful thing to experience and see. Of course, during those times, as a child almost living in the church, most of those experiences have conflicted due to some personal trauma. You have ministers in the church preaching the word of God yet not fully disclosing the facts. They are not living what they preach. My experience as a young girl caused me to question activities in the church in certain towns and states my family, and I traveled.

One experience for me was every Sunday at church, from 8am until almost 9pm, with a break around 1pm to have a big Sunday meal with plenty of desserts with sweet tea and the deacons smoking cigars, cigarettes, and a beer off the church premises. Hilarious when I think about it as I went off to college. During my younger years, I developed early and was on the chubby side, according to the women in the church. Comments like, "*she is a cute fat girl looking like a jelly roll,*" with laughter and touching the body part. I would see them do this to the boys as well. I would ask my mom if we had to stay and have supper at church. The funny thing about this weight challenge and body-shaming was, I was a 9-year-old girl going through a body transition, and they fed us like we weren't going to eat for two weeks. If you didn't eat all the food on your plate, the women in the church would speak harshly about you and to you. Many of the children experienced this unhealthy interaction with food because of these women. The famous words, "Your betta eat all this food because you are wasteful. There are starving children in Africa." *Does the entire continent have starving children?* I thought that but wouldn't dare say it to them. I didn't want missing teeth. If there was a thin woman in the church, most women would make comments about her not eating enough, or no man would want to marry her because she didn't have childbearing hips. GEESH!! Maybe she was naturally thin, perhaps she realizes specific foods could cause health issues mainly if you over-ate all the time, or maybe she liked the way she looked. God forgive her for wanting to look a certain way in her clothes. My issue was the constant judging and smiling in the person's face as if you liked them. Even as a child, I knew that was not the way Jesus would behave. Many adults have unhealthy relationships with food because children grew up being manipulated with food. They were not taught how certain foods can help them have stronger bodies and be better in school. Adults only decide to change when they receive a diagnosis from a doctor when it becomes a health issue or a behavioral problem because of the school's dreaded calls. I am thankful because God revealed to me early while in high school how nutrition and physical activity could help me succeed. I can discuss other issues such as how people in the church communicate with conflicting agendas, but that will be another day. Again, I must remind you; people have flaws, but they should not use the Bible to validate the wrong information they share to hurt, manipulate and prevent others from seeking prosperity.

Respect your body, your temple.

La Tanya

Simple Changes for Your Healthy Mind and Relationships

Power in Words and Knowledge with Action

Whom do you belong to? What is your intent? What is your purpose?

Choose to stay positive and be the strong person God created you to be. We all have faced a dire situation that tried to bring out the worst in us. GOD will work it out for your good, and HE will get the glory.

James 1:5 - If any of you lacks wisdom, let him ask God, who gives generously to all without reproach, and it will be given to him.

I serve with compassion and joy.

LaTonya

Simple Changes for Your Healthy Mind and Relationships

My Journey

My health and knowledge of food have been interesting adventures for 20 years. My first encounter of receiving news of having an unhealthy body was when I was diagnosed with endometriosis, and my physician told me I would have a difficult time conceiving. Most of my life I wanted to be married, have a couple of children and travel the world. Of course, when my doctor gave me this news it saddened me and my life would have a different look. The Lord knew my heart and I believed he would bless me with the life I desired. I prayed to God that whatever he wanted for me I would be pleased and continue to serve in any capacity that would give God glory. When I met my potential husband, we courted for a few months, and soon he asked me to be his bride. My heart was saddened to share the news that I may not be able to bear his children. My God-fearing husband said," GOD told me differently." Whew, that made my heart skip a beat and made me blush. One year after marriage, we decided it was time to expand our family, and I was pregnant immediately. Eighteen months later, I was pregnant again but discovered I had fibroids that caused my menstrual cycle to become heavy and last longer than usual. My husband encouraged me to change my diet and eat greener, exercise more, and stress less. The fibroids shrunk, and I felt normal and healthy. A few years later, my healthy habits took the back seat by

1

indulging in hotdogs, nachos, and all fun summer foods with slacking on my exercise. My fibroids came back with a vengeance, and my body took it hard. Unfortunately, it was too late to go back to eating healthy and my physician failed me by not taking my condition seriously until I was diagnosed with anemia (blood count less than 8) and heart failure due to the extreme blood loss from several months of long menstrual cycles. It was so bad that I had to change my sanitary pads every two hours at work and sometimes, go home to change my clothes during work hours. This medical issue made me feel depressed, weak and like an outcast because I didn't feel comfortable attending events. I could no longer be intimate with my husband. Denying our time together made me angry, and I felt sad for my husband. These multiple fibroids are evil. I felt neglected, ignored, and disrespected by the one person who vowed to make me better. The steroid injection my doctor gave me was supposed to stop the bleeding, only for the bleeding to continue and caused 25 pounds of unnatural weight gain. Another issue to deal with and need to overcome for not just my body, but mentally. The extra weight gain caused joint pain and discomfort. I no longer had the energy to exercise and I felt unattractive to my husband. After surgery to remove the calcified fibroid, my husband and sons were my accountability team to make me healthier and stronger. The fact is God gives us intuition about what is going on with our bodies. We trust what the doctors tell us because they are experts in their field. Sometimes, we trust them too much because man can fail us for their own benefit, which is financial gain.

Health professionals are no longer looking to heal people but finding ways to continue to make money from illnesses. I trusted my OBGYN to give me the best medical advice to rid me of this horrible pain and discomfort. This ailment could have ruined my relationship with my husband, my children, and my advancement in my career. We had the best health coverage money could buy, which allowed my doctor to use these resources for their benefit. Constantly running tests, less invasive procedures to "see" what will make me better. God led me to watch 'Good Morning America' and a doctor spoke about how his colleagues misused medical coverage to gain wealth at the expense of women. His wife was a victim of unnecessary medical procedures because their insurance covered everything under the sun. The other side without insurance are equally or even more neglected. He shared what procedure was commonly used for women with fibroids and what food they should avoid based on the research of a person's race and genetics. During my research and classes, I discovered the medical profession is a trillion-dollar business of keeping sick people sick. There are pharma-companies legally pushing drugs to gain wealth and not heal the unhealthy. Someone shared a post with me last year about the opioids problem. "$$$ Dollars, Dollars, Dollars. It's BONUS time in the neighborhood!!" Purdue Sales Rep. This was focused on poor, working-class labor workers who could not afford to take a day off from work and relied on Oxycontin to treat the pain. I write this workbook to give you information on how I was able to continue to build up my immune system, tone my body, lose the unhealthy weight for my petite body frame, and develop mental clarity about my purpose. Food can promote poor health, but it can also promote healing. If you are dealing with a health issue such as fibroid, it can be the extra motivation you need to start a fibroid-healing diet.

I hope this will bless you and your family~

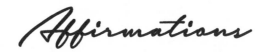

Affirmations

Affirmation for spiritual growth

All my thoughts, words, and actions are divinely guided.

Affirmation for relationship

I attract loving and caring people into my life.

Affirmation for health

I radiate good health.

Affirmation for financial wealth

My income exceeds my expenses.

Remind yourself daily that you are deserving of this and will have the desires of your heart. ♥

Disclaimer:

This content is not intended to be a substitute for professional medical advice, diagnosis, or treatment. Always seek the advice of your physician or other qualified health providers with any questions you may have regarding a medical condition.

Chapter One

FORGET YOUR FIBROIDS

FOOD IS MEDICINE to the body. I did repair my body with changes in how I selected and prepared my meals. With that in mind, here are the top foods for shrinking fibroids that should be a part of your diet. Living with fibroids can be uncomfortable and painful. Doing everything you can at home to benefit your body in the fight against it can help improve your biological system and decrease the symptoms. Make sure to speak with your doctor about managing your fibroids and about any drastic dietary changes. Adding and eliminating certain foods to help regulate estrogen levels in your body may assist in managing fibroids until you can undergo a permanent solution.

Fruits and Vegetables

Fruits and vegetables are very healing not only because of the vitamins and minerals that they contain, but also because of their fiber content which help remove toxins and waste matter from your body promptly before they can cause damage. In addition, increased fiber consumption can help eliminate excess estrogen and help with weight control.

Flaxseed

Flaxseed contains many fibroid healing properties, especially phytoestrogens, which can help replace some of the much stronger and more damaging estrogen produced naturally by the body. This helps to prevent a state of estrogen-dominance which fibroids thrive in.

Legumes

Beans and peas contain properties that can help to promote hormonal balance which is important to shrink fibroids. Legumes are also a rich source of a vital fiber type (soluble fiber) which causes waste matter and toxins, including excessive estrogen, to cling to it on its way out of the body.

Garlic and Onions

These can help to promote gynecological health because they contain antioxidants that prevent free radical damage to healthy cells all over the body, including the pelvic region. Damage from free radicals increases the risk of developing various diseases and conditions.

Cold-water Fish

Deep-sea cold-water fish such as salmon, sardines, tuna, and mackerel should be an essential part of your fibroid healing diet because they are a rich source of essential fatty acids which are anti-inflammatory and can help if you are dealing with fibroids to promote hormone balance.

Gluten-free grains

Carbohydrates are necessary for the energy needed to carry out day-to-day activities, but you need to make sure that you choose the right carbs. Eating grains that do not contain gluten, such as brown rice, wild rice, long grain rice, buckwheat, and millet instead can be more beneficial. These grains also contain many vitamins and minerals that can help to shrink fibroids.

Eggs from free-range birds

Eggs can be very healing because they are not only a great source of protein, but if they are from organically raised birds, their diet is usually supplemented with essential fatty acids, which means that the eggs obtained from these birds will be an excellent source for omega-3 essential fatty acids needed for promoting optimal health.

We had the luxury of raising chickens for years in our backyard. Those eggs were the best I have ever tasted. My weekly gift to my coworkers was sharing our fresh eggs because we were getting almost a dozen per day.

Time to Reflect on How This Changed Your Life

Will this motivate you to make positive changes? If so, how? (write your plans and the steps you will take to make changes)

_____

_____

_____

_____

_____

_____

_____

_____

_____

_____

_____

_____

_____

_____

_____

_____

_____

_____

_____

_____

_____

_____

_____

How did the chapter affect you and share your thoughts on how this information affects your life?

_____

_____

_____

_____

_____

_____

_____

_____

_____

_____

_____

_____

_____

_____

_____

_____

_____

_____

_____

_____

_____

_____

_____

_____

_____

Where do you see yourself in a month or year after you consistently make these changes?

_____

_____

_____

_____

_____

_____

_____

_____

_____

_____

_____

_____

_____

_____

_____

_____

_____

_____

_____

_____

_____

_____

_____

Chapter Two

WHAT ARE UTERINE FIBROIDS?

FIBROIDS ARE ABNORMAL growths in the uterus. They are also called uterine fibroids, myomas, and leiomyomas.

Fibroids are not cancerous or life-threatening, but they can sometimes cause complications and health problems.

Fibroids form in and around the uterine walls. They are made of muscle and other tissues. They may be as tiny as a seed or grow larger than a tennis ball. You may have multiple fibroids or just one.

Doctors don't know exactly what causes fibroids. Being overweight or obese increases the risks, as does having low levels of some types of nutrients.

Prevalence

This condition may also be genetic. You're at higher risk if your mother or sister has fibroids.

Fibroids can cause symptoms and complications such as:

- Pain
- Heavy menstrual bleeding
- Constipation
- Anemia
- Difficulty getting pregnant
- Miscarriages

Chapter Three

HOW TO PREVENT FIBROIDS

WHILE FOODS CAN'T TREAT or prevent fibroids, your daily diet and lifestyle may play a role in reducing your risk. Diet can help balance hormones that may trigger these growths. Certain foods may also help ease fibroid symptoms.

There are several changes you can make that might help reduce your risk for fibroids.

Mediterranean diet

Add plenty of fresh and cooked green vegetables, fresh fruit, legumes, and fish to your plate. A Mediterranean diet is one way to do this. Eating these foods regularly may help lower your risk for fibroids. On the other hand, eating beef, ham, lamb, and other red meat may raise your risk.

Limit alcohol

Drinking any type of alcohol may increase your risk for fibroids. This can happen because alcohol raises the level of hormones needed for fibroids to grow. Alcohol may also trigger inflammation. A study found that women who drank one or more beers a day increased their risk by more than 50 percent.

Estrogen is a hormone essential for healthy fertility in both women and men. However, too much estrogen can make the growth of fibroids worse. Many treatments for fibroids work by lowering estrogen levels. Other ways to balance estrogen levels include:

Losing weight. Obesity increases the risk for fibroids. Fat cells make more estrogen, so losing weight may help prevent or slow the growth of fibroids.

Avoiding hormone-disrupting chemicals. Natural and synthetic chemicals can throw off your endocrine balance, raising estrogen levels. These chemicals can leach into your body through skin and food. Avoid or limit encountering chemicals found in:

- fertilizers
- pesticides
- plastics such as BPA
- nonstick coatings on cookware
- dyes
- paints

Healthy blood pressure. Research shows that a high number of women with severe fibroids also have high blood pressure. More research is needed to find out if there's a link.

Balancing blood pressure is vital for your overall health. Try these tips:

- Avoid added salt. Flavor food with herbs and other spices instead
- Limit high sodium-processed and packaged foods
- Check your blood pressure daily with a home monitor
- Exercise regularly
- Lose weight, especially around the waist
- Avoid or limit alcohol intake
- Increase potassium by eating most plants at each meal
- Quit smoking and avoid secondhand smoke
- If you have high blood pressure, take medication as prescribed
- See your doctor for regular checkups

Vitamin D may help reduce your risk of fibroids by almost 60 percent. Your body makes this "sunshine vitamin" naturally when your skin's exposed to sunlight. If you have darker skin or live-in cooler climates, you're more likely to be deficient.

Supplements can help raise your levels, along with foods such as:

- egg yolks
- fortified orange juice
- fatty fish such as salmon, tuna, and mackerel
- cod liver oil

Eating brightly colored fruits and vegetables is suitable for your general health. Consuming a variety of red, yellow, and orange foods will provide rich antioxidants. Dark greens are also nutrient-dense and will provide healthful benefits. These nutrients may help protect you from diseases, including some cancers.

I. Best Foods to Eat

1) Organic foods
2) Green leafy vegetables
3) Beta-carotene rich foods (such as carrots and sweet potatoes)
4) Food high in iron (such as grass-fed beef and legumes)
5) Flaxseeds
6) Whole grains

II. Foods to Shrink Fibroids

1) Fruits and Vegetables
2) Flaxseed
3) Legumes
4) Garlic and Onions
5) Cold-water Fish
6) Gluten-free grains.
7) Eggs from free-range birds

III. Foods to Avoid for Fibroids

These foods should be eliminated from your diet to help regulate estrogen levels in your body. These were the foods that caused the fibroids to come back, causing more health issues for me. Don't misunderstand me. I have ice cream maybe twice a year.

• If possible, any foods that increase estrogen levels in your body should be avoided. Red meat, alcohol, animal fats, cheese, cream, butter, ice cream, and chocolate have all been shown to raise estrogen levels. The fat from turkey and chicken should also be trimmed before cooking.

• Low-fat milk should be swapped for whole milk.

• Artificial sweeteners should also be eliminated; remember to read the ingredient list on the food label.

• Soy products have been shown to increase estrogen levels, so cut these out as well.

• Avoid storing food in plastic containers. Studies have shown that plastic can leech into the food from the containers, which will influence your body's estrogen levels when consumed.

- Table sugar
- Glucose
- Dextrose
- Maltose
- Corn syrup
- High fructose corn syrup
- White bread, rice, pasta, and flour
- Soda and sugary drinks

IV. Foods to Fight Fibroids

• Cruciferous vegetables help the liver detox. Broccoli, cabbage, bok choy, kale, turnips, watercress, radish, and arugula are great choices. Avoid overcooking these vegetables so that they retain most of their nutrients.

• Foods to help detoxify your body are also

recommended. Garlic, carrots, beets, and drinking plenty of water will help with detoxification.

• Foods that contain carotenes should be added to your diet for fibroids. Apricots, sweet potato, cantaloupe, carrots, pumpkin, and spinach are all-sufficient sources.

• Eat foods containing vitamin E, like almonds, wheat germ, hazelnuts, and cod liver oil.

• Natural anti-inflammatory foods can help as well. Pineapple and fresh rosemary have been shown to help decrease inflammation.

• An antioxidant called polyphenol, which is found in green tea, can help counteract estrogen effects.

• Consider taking a multivitamin every day. Look for one that has 100% daily value for vitamins: B1 (thiamin), B2 (riboflavin), B3 (niacin), B12, and B6. Vitamins C, D, E, and folic acid should also be included, and a max of 15,000 IUs of beta-carotene (vitamin A).

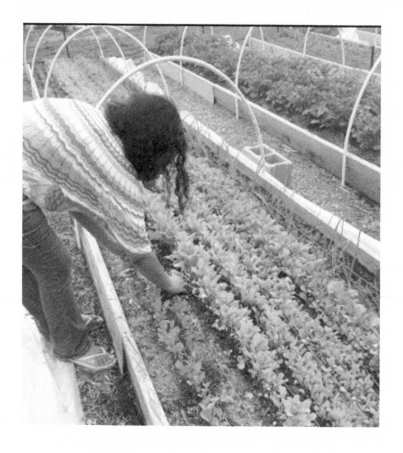

Time to Reflect on How This Changed Your Life

Will this motivate you to make positive changes? If so, how? (write your plans and the steps you will take to make changes)

_____

_____

_____

_____

_____

_____

_____

_____

_____

_____

_____

_____

_____

_____

_____

_____

_____

_____

_____

_____

_____

_____

_____

How did the chapter affect you and share your thoughts on how this information affects your life?

_____

_____

_____

_____

_____

_____

_____

_____

_____

_____

_____

_____

_____

_____

_____

_____

_____

_____

_____

_____

_____

_____

_____

_____

_____

_____

Where do you see yourself in a month or year after you consistently make these changes?

_____

_____

_____

_____

_____

_____

_____

_____

_____

_____

_____

_____

_____

_____

_____

_____

_____

_____

_____

_____

_____

_____

_____

_____

_____

Chapter Four

Cooking time

Breakfast

- Dairy products, such as almond milk and Greek yogurt(unflavored)
- Egg yolks
- Fortified breakfast cereals: Post Great Grains Crunchy Pecan, Kashi GO Lean Original Fiber
- One Honey Clusters and Food for Life Ezekiel 4:9 Sprouted Whole Grain Cereal

Lunch

Spinach salad with diced beets and flaxseeds and a side of tuna or sardines.

or

Romaine lettuce, arugula, and radishes salad, chia seeds eggs.

Dinner

Broccoli, wild rice and mackerel prepared with garlic and onions.

or

Cabbage, salmon, wild rice

Snack

Berries, yogurt and honey

or

Banana and melted dark chocolate.

Easy Beverage

Pear Frost with Ginger

2 cups of pears peeled and chopped

1 cup of apple juice

1tspp fresh ginger root, grated

1 cup of crushed ice

1. Combine
2. Pour over crushed ice. Serve with stainless steel or bamboo straws. Let's be kind to the Earth.

Always drink water and no alcohol. Be kind to your liver and kidneys. These are your staple foods for a healthy gut and immune system.

Brown rice, wild rice, long grain rice, buckwheat, millet, and flaxseeds replace some of the much stronger and more damaging estrogen produced naturally by the body, which can help prevent estrogen dominance that fibroids thrive in.

- Oily fish, such as salmon, herring, and sardines
- Arugula
- Bok choy
- Broccoli
- Brussels sprouts
- Cabbage
- Cauliflower
- Collard greens
- Horseradish
- Radishes
- Rutabagas
- Turnips
- Watercress
- Wasabi

Time to Reflect on How This Changed Your Life

Will this motivate you to make positive changes? If so, how? (write your plans and the steps you will take to make changes)

_____

_____

_____

_____

_____

_____

_____

_____

_____

_____

_____

_____

_____

_____

_____

_____

_____

_____

_____

_____

_____

_____

_____

_____

How did the chapter affect you and share your thoughts on how this information affects your life?

_____

_____

_____

_____

_____

_____

_____

_____

_____

_____

_____

_____

_____

_____

_____

_____

_____

_____

_____

_____

_____

_____

_____

_____

_____

_____

Where do you see yourself in a month or year after you consistently make these changes?

_____

_____

_____

_____

_____

_____

_____

_____

_____

_____

_____

_____

_____

_____

_____

_____

_____

_____

_____

_____

_____

_____

_____

_____

Chapter Five

Messy MS Multiple Sclerosis

THE CAUSE OF MULTIPLE sclerosis is unknown. It's an autoimmune disease in which the body's immune system attacks its own tissues. This immune system malfunction destroys the fatty substance that coats and protects nerve fibers in the brain and spinal cord, resulting in nerve damage and disrupt in communication between the brain and body.

Multiple sclerosis causes many various symptoms, including vision loss, pain, fatigue, and impaired coordination. The symptoms, severity, and duration can vary from person to person. Some people may be symptom-free most of their lives, while others can have severe, chronic symptoms that never go away.

Physical therapy and medications that suppress the immune system can help with symptoms and slow disease progression. It's also common for people with MS to gain weight due to their symptoms. It's essential to try and reach a moderate weight and maintain it. Being overweight or underweight can worsen MS symptoms. We will discuss the foods that can help with slowing the progression of this disease.

Time to Reflect on How This Changed Your Life

Will this motivate you to make positive changes? If so, how? (write your plans and the steps you will take to make changes)

_____

_____

_____

_____

_____

_____

_____

_____

_____

_____

_____

_____

_____

_____

_____

_____

_____

_____

_____

_____

_____

_____

_____

_____

How did the chapter affect you and share your thoughts on how this information affects your life?

_____

_____

_____

_____

_____

_____

_____

_____

_____

_____

_____

_____

_____

_____

_____

_____

_____

_____

_____

_____

_____

_____

_____

_____

_____

_____

_____

Where do you see yourself in a month or year after you consistently make these changes?

_____

_____

_____

_____

_____

_____

_____

_____

_____

_____

_____

_____

_____

_____

_____

_____

_____

_____

_____

_____

_____

_____

_____

_____

Chapter Six

Move away MS with these tasty foods.

FATTY FISH — such as trout, salmon, tuna, mackerel, and herring (including sardines) — are good sources of omega-3 fatty acids. Omega-3s are widely understood to have cardiovascular benefits, and they appear to help block the body's inflammatory response.

When it comes to direct benefits for MS, the results are less clear-cut. It shows that omega-3s might have a small effect in promoting the rebuilding of myelin, the coating on nerve fibers that are attacked in MS.

At least a couple of studies, including in April 2018, in the journal Neurology, have found that a higher intake of fatty fish may lower a person's risk of developing MS.

Fruits and vegetables are rich in phytochemicals and antioxidants, substances that may help reduce inflammation. An anti-inflammatory diet should include foods like tomatoes, leafy greens such as spinach and kale, and fruits like strawberries, blueberries, cherries, and oranges.

There's some evidence that consuming these foods could be beneficial for MS. In a study published in January 2018, in the journal Neurology, a diet rich in fruits and vegetables was found to correlate with less disability and lower symptom severity in people with MS, including less fatigue, pain, cognitive impairment, and depression.

However, there were other dietary factors in that study that make it unclear how much fruits and vegetables were responsible for the results.

Turmeric is a vibrant yellow, fragrant spice that grows as a rhizome (underground stem). It can be used fresh, but it's most widely available in its dried and powdered form.

The most widely studied molecule in turmeric, known as curcumin, has been shown to have numerous potentially beneficial effects in the human body — some of which could be especially relevant to MS. As noted in a research review published in January 2017, in the Journal of Cellular Physiology, curcumin can affect various cells in your immune system which may decrease the severity of diseases stemming from an immune-system response.

Ginger is another rhizome with a potent, spicy flavor. Like turmeric, it can be used fresh or dried and powdered.

Fresh ginger and ginger extracts are believed to contain several different anti-inflammatory compounds. One of these, 10-gingerol, is believed to be the most important in reducing neuroinflammation — inflammation in the brain or spinal cord.

There's provisional evidence that extra-virgin olive oil — and components in it known as phenols — may help prevent the inflammatory processes involved in a variety of chronic diseases.

In fact, research found that out of 30 studies enrolling over 3,000 people, consuming olive oil was associated with a pronounced decrease in two inflammatory markers, C-reactive protein, and interleukin-6. There was also strong evidence that consuming olive oil resulted in improved blood vessel function.

Walnuts are a good source of omega-3s and other healthy unsaturated fats. Like some other types of nuts, they're also packed with antioxidants, fiber, and magnesium, all of which have important roles in regulating inflammation.

Consuming walnuts has been shown to reduce levels of two blood markers involved in the inflammatory response.

Meal planning

Spinach Catalan

10 cups of fresh spinach leaves

1/3 pine nuts

3 cloves of crushed garlic

½ cup raisins golden

1/3 cup olive oil

1. Place raisin in a bowl with hot water, cover for 10 minutes before draining.
2. Heat garlic in a sauté pan in olive oil medium, heat until golden, then remove.
3. Add the spinach to the infused garlic oil and cook for 3 minutes.
4. Add the raisin and pine nuts and cook for 2 minutes.
5. Season with salt and pepper.
6. Serve while hot.

Broccoli Egg cups

3 cups chopped broccoli florets

2 cups shredded cheddar cheese

8 large eggs beaten.

1 tsp basil

½ cup low-fat milk

½ tsp Dijon mustard

Salt and pepper

1. Lightly oil muffin tin and preheat oven to 350 F
2. Mix eggs, milk mustard, basil salt, and pepper in a bowl
3. Divide the broccoli and cheese in each muffin tin section
4. Pour the egg mixture over the broccoli in each section of the muffin tin
5. Bake for 30 minutes
6. Let it cool and serve. Great for breakfast on the go and a late snack

Testimony

Patty S of St Louis has MS for more than 9 years and learned that water was the big thing for her to maintain a healthy weight and stay cool. Some people with MS experience a worsening of their symptoms when they become very hot because of hot weather, exercise, or taking a hot shower. If you're sensitive to heat, it's important to stay hydrated so your body can naturally cool itself down with perspiration.

Time to Reflect on How This Changed Your Life

Will this motivate you to make positive changes? If so, how? (write your plans and the steps you will take to make changes)

_____

_____

_____

_____

_____

_____

_____

_____

_____

_____

_____

_____

_____

_____

_____

_____

_____

_____

_____

_____

_____

_____

_____

How did the chapter affect you and share your thoughts on how this information affects your life?

_____

_____

_____

_____

_____

_____

_____

_____

_____

_____

_____

_____

_____

_____

_____

_____

_____

_____

_____

_____

_____

_____

_____

_____

Where do you see yourself in a month or year after you consistently make these changes?

_____

_____

_____

_____

_____

_____

_____

_____

_____

_____

_____

_____

_____

_____

_____

_____

_____

_____

_____

_____

_____

_____

_____

_____

_____

Chapter Seven

HEAL MY BODY WITH NATURE'S MEDICINE

(while filling my tummy and eating tasty food.)

WE TALK ABOUT EATING healthy and having a healthy diet, but do we really know what that looks like? You must have an abundance of fruit and whole grains, a moderate amount of "good fats and lean, yes, lean protein, which will help prevent and control life-threatening diseases such as heart disease and diabetes. Did you know certain foods have an immediate benefit to tame common health problems such as headaches and insomnia? So, the next time you experience one of the conditions below, consider heading to your kitchen before you open your medicine cabinet.

I. Sip away headaches

Whether you have headaches frequently or occasionally, the first thing to do if you get one is drinking a tall glass of water or two. Dehydration is a common cause of headaches, so water may address the pain right away.

Having a snack with a combination of carbs, protein, and healthy fat may also help because it prevents blood sugar dips, which can trigger headaches. A good combo snack is an apple with a handful of walnuts.

However, for some people, caffeine can set off a headache, so if that happens to you, skip the coffee. But if you experience migraines, be aware that food reputed to trigger those headaches—aged cheese, cured meats, chocolate, artificial sweeteners, MSG, and soy—are to blame much less often than you might think.

If you suspect that certain foods trigger your headaches, keeping a food diary can pinpoint dietary culprits.

II. Ban nausea with a spice

Ginger has been extensively studied as a potential remedy for nausea, especially during chemotherapy and pregnancy. It seems to help by moving food out of the stomach quickly and turning off neurotransmitters such as serotonin that can contribute to nausea.

Make yourself some ginger tea, steep 1½ teaspoons of freshly grated ginger in 1½ cups of boiling water (add honey if you like). Let it sit for 10 minutes, then strain the ginger out before drinking.

And do not think you have to stick with rice and dry toast after a bout of nausea. William Chey, M.D., a gastroenterologist, and professor of medicine and nutrition at the University of Michigan, Ann Arbor, says evidence does not support long-standing advice to eat only bland foods. He recommends small, frequent meals rich in protein, especially chicken and fish, and vegetable proteins.

"Red meat is hard to digest," Chey says. "There are other proteins that seem to move through the stomach more quickly."

"Plus, they don't cause the same gastric sensations that fats do," he adds. Fats can make the stomach overly sensitive, leading to pain, fullness, and nausea.

III. Nighty, night, snack away your insomnia

Some people suggest sipping warm milk for insomnia because it contains tryptophan, an amino acid converted to serotonin, which will relax you, and melatonin, which promotes sleep. But studies have not proved that.

"It might help some people because it's a calming ritual, not because of the tryptophan."

A healthy snack will include two kiwis an hour before bedtime. A 2016 review of studies published in Advances in Nutrition concluded that the fruit may promote sleep because it's a rich source of folate, a B-vitamin that may help the brain produce sleep-inducing chemicals.

Kiwi's high antioxidant content may also be a factor. Those plant-based chemicals combat oxidative stress— cell and DNA damage from factors such as exposure to the sun, smoking, and pollution—which has been linked to sleep problems. But more research is needed on the kiwi-sleep connection.

IV. Goodbye heartburn with fruit

The typical dietary advice for fighting heartburn and gastroesophageal reflux disorder (GERD) is to eat smaller, more frequent meals, skip spicy foods, and avoid eating or drinking within 3 to 4 hours of bedtime.

The problem is that it only helps reduce the likelihood of future attacks. Once the burning sensation strikes, try having a banana. Some research suggests that the fruit may act as a natural antacid.

Another remedy: Chew sugarless gum. Studies have found that it may decrease reflux after a meal.

Long-term, consider cutting back on your consumption of sugars. A 16-week study of obese women, published this year in the journal Alimentary Pharmacology and Therapeutics, found that reducing refined carbohydrates, mainly sucrose (table sugar), eliminated symptoms in those who complained of GERD at the start of the trial.

V. Don't starve, but feed the cold

No foods are a proven remedy to shorten a cold, but some may help ease sneezing, a sore throat, and a stuffy nose caused by inflammation. "Your body needs more antioxidants during the cold season, so eating more fruit and vegetables is key to feeling your best. "

What about chicken soup? A study published in the Chest Journal many years ago found that chicken soup made with sweet potato, turnips, and other healthy ingredients did a better job of reducing inflammation than plain chicken broth. (Store-bought brands worked, too.) Soup is also hydrating, which helps your lymph system flush out the virus.

But you may want to avoid sugars when you have a cold. "There's some research showing sugar weakens the activity of certain [virus-fighting] white blood cells. Plus, you need a lot of nutrients to keep your body strong during a cold or flu, and sugary foods take the place of healthier options."

VI. Mental clarity. I can see better now

Using high-quality herbs and spices will provide not only the best taste but also the best healing. Grow your own herbs if possible or buy organic spices. Let color and scent be your guides–the more vibrant and aromatic, the better. Store them in a cool, dark area and replace them once a year or when they fade in color or aroma. Your food will become delicious medicine–a recipe for wellness and productivity. Bon Appetit!

Whether you consume these herbs in tea form or use them to spice up meals, you'll reap the rewarding benefits.

Sage has been used since medieval times to improve memory and to treat dementia. A clinical study of Alzheimer's patients found sage to be effective for improving their cognition. Sage also has antioxidant, antimicrobial, astringent, and antispasmodic properties.

Herbalists in the 1820s recognized this herb's potential as a tranquilizer and sedative. Valerian may help relieve sleep difficulties, thereby naturally improve cognition, memory, and concentration. The herb's tranquilizing properties also improve concentration by relieving stress.

Turmeric, a common ingredient in curries is a super-hero herb. It relieves inflammatory conditions like skin problems, dementia, pain, and arthritis. Studies now suggest it may be useful in battling cancer and preventing Alzheimer's disease. Turmeric is revered in India, where the rate of Alzheimer's is low compared with the Western world rate. Now that is something to consider!

Rosemary has excellent antioxidant properties that help the body fight free radicals–molecules responsible for aging. Boosting brain function, rosemary also treats poor memory, mental fogginess, and fatigue. This herb has also been known to increase alertness.

Garlic, though not an herb, improves the flavor and aroma of multiple dishes and is used world-wide. As one of the oldest known cultivated crops, garlic has been used medicinally since ancient times. Eating this powerful antibiotic is an effective way to detoxify and treat illness. Garlic clears up congestion, reduces blood pressure and cholesterol, and balances the flora of the gut. Consuming raw garlic is great for your overall health.

VII. For my sensitive sinus sisters

Vitamins and minerals — colorful fruits and vegetables — like apricots, cantaloupe, strawberries, red and green peppers, kale, parsley, and broccoli — get high praise from the scientists working on sinus healers world-wide. They contain lots of vitamin C which is known to fend off colds, allergies, and sinus infections. You also need vitamin A to keep your mucous membranes healthy. If you eat carrots, sweet potatoes, mangoes, winter squash, you will get lots of beta carotene, which your body converts to vitamin A. Zinc, found in seafood, dark turkey meat, and black beans, helps change beta carotene to vitamin A. It also helps build up your immunity and reduces the risk of respiratory infections that can lead to colds. Vitamin E is also strongly recommended for preventing allergies and sinusitis, and its power is doubled when you get selenium with it. Whole grains grown in enriched soils can provide you with both these nutrients.

Ginger-garlic — The stinky compound in garlic, allicin, kills fungi and bacteria and gives your immune system a much-needed boost.

Water — Keeping your mucous membranes moist will increase your resistance to infection and allow your sinuses to drain more easily. So, drink lots of water — even more than the recommended 8 glasses of water a day, especially if you exercise a lot. For variety, include herbal teas, natural fruit juices diluted 50 percent with water or thin soups but choose products with less salt and no added sugar. Avoid drinking too much coffee, tea and cola as these drinks contribute to dehydration and mucous production.

VIII. Don't believe the hype about sweets

You may think of milk, sweets, sweet beverages as comfort foods. Still, if you are battling sinusitis, they will add to your discomfort as the protein in milk tends to increase and thicken mucous secretions. Please avoid milk and dairy products, especially at the time of sinus attack.

Eating this will help

Apricots, strawberries, parsley, mangoes, cantaloupe, kale, sweet potatoes, broccoli, black beans, whole wheat bread.

This is a No-No

Dairy products, sugar in large amounts, wine, yes, even red wine, alcohol, etc.

IX. Happiness over depression

Fresh produce like kale, berries, and mushrooms can curb symptoms of depression.

Among all the strategies to safeguard my mental health, eating the right foods ties for first (with getting adequate sleep) as the most important. Recently, I did some substantial research on which foods promote sanity and which ones send an alarm to your limbic system (emotion center) and cause inflammation. I decided to eliminate gluten, dairy, caffeine, and sugar from my diet. I also started eating fresh produce throughout my day, and my body felt light and energetic.

I try to eat cucumbers, spinach, avocados, and beets in my salad each day for lunch because they contain lots of folic acids and alpha-lipoic acid, both of which are good for fighting depression. In most of the studies, about one-third of depression patients were deficient in folate.

Folic acid can prevent an excess of homocysteine — which restricts the production of important neurotransmitters like serotonin, dopamine, and norepinephrine — from forming in the body. Alpha-lipoic acid keeps coming up as I read more about nutrition and the brain, so I have begun to take it as a supplement, as well. It helps the body convert glucose into energy and I have made the commitment to hit the grocery store a few times a week.

As a result, I feel more emotionally resilient and less vulnerable to the impact of stress and drama on my mood.

Here are some of the foods I eat every day to feel good. They provide the nutrients my body needs to fight off inflammation in my brain, which leads to depression.

If you were to choose the healthiest food of all, the most nutrient-dense item available to us to eat, it would be dark, leafy greens, no contest. Spinach. Kale. Swiss chard. Greens, beans, onions, mushrooms, berries, seeds with the most powerful immune-boosting and anti-cancer effects.

These foods help prevent the cancerous transformation of normal cells and keep the body armed and ready to attack any precancerous or cancerous cells that may arise. Leafy greens fight against all kinds of inflammation. Severe depression has been linked with brain inflammation. Leafy greens are especially important because they contain oodles of vitamins A, C, E, and K, minerals, and phytochemicals.

Walnuts are one of the richest plant sources of omega-3 fatty acids, and numerous studies have demonstrated how omega-3 fatty acids support brain function and reduce depression symptoms. Blueberries, raspberries, strawberries, and blackberries are some of the highest antioxidant foods available to us. I try to have a variety for breakfast in the morning. Antioxidants are like DNA repairmen. They go around fixing your cells and preventing them from getting cancer and other illnesses. Here are two good reasons why mushrooms are good for your mental health. First, their chemical properties oppose insulin, which helps lower blood sugar levels, evening out your mood. They also are like a probiotic in that they promote healthy gut bacteria. And since the nerve cells in our gut manufacture 80 to 90 percent of our body's serotonin — the critical neurotransmitter that keeps us sane — we can't afford to not pay attention to our intestinal health.

You won't find this item on most lists of mood foods. Onions and all allium vegetables (garlic, leeks, chives, shallots, and spring onions) have been associated with a decreased risk of several cancers.

"Eating onions and garlic frequently is associated with a reduced risk of cancers of the digestive tract. These vegetables also contain high concentrations of anti-inflammatory flavonoid antioxidants that contribute to their anti-cancer properties. Again, suppose you consider the relationship between your digestive tract and your brain. In that case, it is understandable why a food that can prevent cancers of the gut would also benefit your mood.

Beans are good for the heart. They can act as anti-diabetes and weight-loss foods. They are good for my mood because my body (and yours) digests them slowly, which stabilizes blood sugar levels. Any food that assists me in evening out my blood sugar levels is my friend. They are the one starch that I allow myself, so they help mitigate my craving for bread and other processed grains on top of a salad.

When I'm close to reaching for potato chips or any kind of comfort food, I allow myself a few handfuls of sunflower seeds or any other type of seed I can find in our kitchen.

Flaxseeds, hemp seeds, and chia seeds are especially good for your mood because they are rich in omega-3 fatty acids. Not only do seeds add their own spectrum of unique disease-fighting substances to the dietary landscape, but the fat in seeds increases the absorption of protective nutrients in vegetables eaten at the same meal."

Indeed, an apple a day could — if eaten with the rest of these foods — keep the psychiatrist away, at least for periods. Like berries, apples are high in antioxidants, which can help to prevent and repair oxidation damage and inflammation on the cellular level. They are also full of soluble fiber, which balances blood sugar swings.

Time to Reflect on How This Changed Your Life

Will this motivate you to make positive changes? If so, how? (write your plans and the steps you will take to make changes)

_____

_____

_____

_____

_____

_____

_____

_____

_____

_____

_____

_____

_____

_____

_____

_____

_____

_____

_____

_____

_____

_____

_____

_____

How did the chapter affect you and share your thoughts on how this information affects your life?

_____

_____

_____

_____

_____

_____

_____

_____

_____

_____

_____

_____

_____

_____

_____

_____

_____

_____

_____

_____

_____

_____

_____

_____

_____

Where do you see yourself in a month or year after you consistently make these changes?

_____

_____

_____

_____

_____

_____

_____

_____

_____

_____

_____

_____

_____

_____

_____

_____

_____

_____

_____

_____

_____

_____

_____

_____

Chapter Eight

SPICES FOR HEALTH

Garlic – Natural antibiotic, immune booster, lowers blood pressure

Thyme-Reduces headaches and mucous

Fennel-Appetite suppressants, digestive helper

Ginger- Immune booster, settles stomach

Mustard Seeds-Aids in breaking down fat

Parsley- May prevent cancer cell multiplication, freshens breath

Turmeric- Natural antibiotic, anti-inflammatory, aids in skin health

Chive- Respiratory and prostate health

Celery Seed- Natural diuretic water pill

Cinnamon- Boost glucose metabolism, diabetes prevention

Cayenne Pepper- Stabilize blood sugar, speeds metabolism, warms the body, blood pressure equalizer

Oregano- natural anti-viral, immune booster, heals skin

Evaluated by the FDA; consult with your physician before self-medicating

Time to Reflect on How This Changed Your Life

Will this motivate you to make positive changes? If so, how? (write your plans and the steps you will take to make changes)

_____

_____

_____

_____

_____

_____

_____

_____

_____

_____

_____

_____

_____

_____

_____

_____

_____

_____

_____

_____

_____

_____

_____

How did the chapter affect you and share your thoughts on how this information affects your life?

_____

_____

_____

_____

_____

_____

_____

_____

_____

_____

_____

_____

_____

_____

_____

_____

_____

_____

_____

_____

_____

_____

_____

_____

_____

_____

Where do you see yourself in a month or year after you consistently make these changes?

_____

_____

_____

_____

_____

_____

_____

_____

_____

_____

_____

_____

_____

_____

_____

_____

_____

_____

_____

_____

_____

_____

_____

_____

_____

Chapter Nine

Natural Oils/Aromatherapy to heal body and spiritual wounds

TAKE A BREAK and reflect on yourself. You are an extraordinary individual.

Legend has it that frankincense has been used to support healthy bodily function for thousands of years. During biblical times, frankincense was said to be valued even more than gold. One study indicated that the essential oil can indeed help improve memory retention and sharpen the mind.

Vetiver is a thicker oil that carries an earthy fragrance. It has powerful calming and grounding effects on emotions, making it a popular oil in massage therapy. It has been shown to reduce stress in sleep-deprived rats and is often used in humans to promote restful sleep and aid in recovery from emotional turmoil.

Citrus oils like lemon are very uplifting to the mind and body. Lemon, when used aromatically, promotes physical energy and purification. Its invigorating fragrance is warming, and certain studies support the use of lemon essential oil for reducing stress and boosting mood and focus.

Peppermint is a popular oil that stimulates the mind to help support memory, focus, concentration, and mental performance. There was a study on more than 20 participants. Those who ingested a higher concentration of peppermint essential oil reported less mental fatigue after cognitively demanding tasks.

For worried, anxious thoughts:

- Vetiver
- Lavender
- Frankincense
- Ylang Ylang
- Clary Sage

To elevate mood and increase vitality:

- Lavender
- Hawaiian Sandalwood
- Ylang Ylang
- Wild Orange

When choosing essential oils, it's important to do your research and make sure you're getting therapeutic-grade oils that are made using the purest ingredients. When you've chosen your oils, diffuse 3 to 6 drops of them in your home or office using a diffuser, inhale a couple of drops from the bottle, or place a few drops of a skin-safe oil in an Epsom bath salt for the ultimate at-home spa treatment.

Time to Reflect on How This Changed Your Life

Will this motivate you to make positive changes? If so, how? (write your plans and the steps you will take to make changes)

_____

_____

_____

_____

_____

_____

_____

_____

_____

_____

_____

_____

_____

_____

_____

_____

_____

_____

_____

_____

_____

_____

_____

How did the chapter affect you and share your thoughts on how this information affects your life?

_____

_____

_____

_____

_____

_____

_____

_____

_____

_____

_____

_____

_____

_____

_____

_____

_____

_____

_____

_____

_____

_____

Where do you see yourself in a month or year after you consistently make these changes?

_____

_____

_____

_____

_____

_____

_____

_____

_____

_____

_____

_____

_____

_____

_____

_____

_____

_____

_____

_____

_____

_____

_____

_____

_____

Chapter Ten

FASTING FOR FREEDOM AND LASTING BENEFITS

A GROUP OF CANADIAN scientists recently studied fruit flies' brain activity and found that acute fasting directly influences the stability of neuronal circuits, a type of wiring that dictates the flow of information in the brain and nervous system. According to their paper, the cellular stress and lack of nutrition catalyzed by fasting block the neurons' synaptic activity that normally occurs in the brain, which means that the brain slows down.

And although a brain "slowing down" sounds undesirable, it may be beneficial for brain health. The overactive synaptic activity has been associated with diseases like Parkinson's, Alzheimer's, and other degenerative diseases. So, in a way, when we slow down our brain activity, it's possible that we are protecting the organ by allowing it to recharge.

Results also showed an increase in ketone bodies due to fasting, which are neuroprotective compounds, guarding brain cells against degenerating to the point of disease. The ketogenic (low-carb and high-fat) diet has been used since the 1920s as an extremely effective treatment for epilepsy, even though the mechanism by which it works was mostly unknown.

Close to 40 percent of Americans are deficient in vitamin B12, which can result in fatigue, memory loss, mental fogginess, and even depressed mood. Vitamin B12 helps with the normal functioning of the nervous system, including the brain. People with higher levels of vitamin B12 seem to have less brain shrinkage as they get older.

Taking vitamin B12 when you are deficient can be helpful to address memory, mental clarity, overall energy, and depressed mood. However, if you are not deficient in vitamin B12 (a blood test will tell you), it may not be as helpful.

If you have only three minutes in the morning to dedicate, I highly suggest you first, express your gratitude for another day and then your yoga practice, this simple exercise is the one I recommend most to eliminate brain fog and fatigue—two of the most common symptoms of thyroid disorders and hormone imbalances.

Testimony

Jaime A. Texas

Depression runs in my family and being a compulsive eater made my emotional state even worse. I admit that the first day I tried to fast was hard. Drinking water, trying to keep busy so I didn't eat and staying on track with the food selection. Day two was easier and day three became a challenge again, but I started to realize food was preventing me from actually working on meaningful projects. Reading, meditating, and listening to music helped.

Time to Reflect on How This Changed Your Life

Will this motivate you to make positive changes? If so, how? (write your plans and the steps you will take to make changes)

_____

_____

_____

_____

_____

_____

_____

_____

_____

_____

_____

_____

_____

_____

_____

_____

_____

_____

_____

_____

_____

_____

_____

_____

How did the chapter affect you and share your thoughts on how this information affects your life?

_____

_____

_____

_____

_____

_____

_____

_____

_____

_____

_____

_____

_____

_____

_____

_____

_____

_____

_____

_____

_____

_____

_____

_____

Where do you see yourself in a month or year after you consistently make these changes?

_____

_____

_____

_____

_____

_____

_____

_____

_____

_____

_____

_____

_____

_____

_____

_____

_____

_____

_____

_____

_____

_____

Chapter Eleven

WAKE THE BODY, MOVE WITH EASE AND CONSISTENCY

My weekly routine

I personally enjoy the yoga position of cat-cow, known as spinal flexion, which increases the circulation of the spinal fluid. This contributes to greater mental clarity because all 26 vertebrae receive stimulation, and all the body's energy centers get a wake-up call.

What should you do to take care of yourself? It is easy, and others will follow your lead. Your physical wellness is especially important, but others may say mental is the top.

1. Adjust the order to your situation. Habits and goals.
2. Physical get 6-8 hours of restful sleep.
3. Enjoy more fruit and vegetables every day. Makes the tummy happy and the skin glow.

4. Mind your business, practice mindful activities every day for 10-15 minutes. I like coloring, so do children, see how happy they are when they finish?

5. Technology makes life easier, yet it has a time and place, not in bed or first thing in the morning.

6. Do not let your emotions rule your behavior. Practice positive self-talk.

7. Spiritual growth is gold. Read the Bible, pray, be one with nature. Weekends are perfect.

8. Relationships are wonderful, yet practice setting limits with others when you feel overwhelmed by saying NO. (Disclaimer: Watch your tone.)

9. We need our job, but we need to manage the energy that can be too much to handle.

Take these simple tips and see how it works for you. If you are living with others, share with them to make your home more positive.

Testimony

Tiffany F

I was able to make a few changes, such as waking up earlier to meditate and stretch each morning. This helps my day go much smoother. The traffic didn't bother me as much because I was not in a rush and had time to reflect on gratitude.

Time to Reflect on How This Changed Your Life

Will this motivate you to make positive changes? If so, how? (write your plans and the steps you will take to make changes)

_____

_____

_____

_____

_____

_____

_____

_____

_____

_____

_____

_____

_____

_____

_____

_____

_____

_____

_____

_____

_____

_____

_____

How did the chapter affect you and share your thoughts on how this information affects your life?

_____

_____

_____

_____

_____

_____

_____

_____

_____

_____

_____

_____

_____

_____

_____

_____

_____

_____

_____

_____

_____

_____

_____

_____

Where do you see yourself in a month or year after you consistently make these changes?

_____

_____

_____

_____

_____

_____

_____

_____

_____

_____

_____

_____

_____

_____

_____

_____

_____

_____

_____

_____

_____

_____

_____

_____

_____

Chapter Twelve

LET US BE HEALTHY

Fruits: eat whole fruit instead of fruit (sugar) juices. They are great snacks (not snickers).

Vegetables: Choose red, orange, and dark green (they will fill you up and give you energy).

Grains: Whole grain will keep you moving literally.

Protein: Not just meat, eggs, beans, and tofu will have your muscle nice and strong.

Water, Water, Water is like gold!! It keeps the entire body functioning.

Dried chamomile flowers have been used for centuries, and there is research suggesting the tea helps an upset stomach. The flowers contain compounds called flavonoids that may help reduce inflammation and pain.

How to eat it
Make a healthy "hot toddy" with hot chamomile tea, honey, and sliced lemon.

When you have a cold, a little fennel is your friend. Inside this licorice-flavored vegetable are compounds that may help loosen chest mucus and soothe a sore throat. **Fennel** is also a good source of potassium, essential in regulating the fluid balance in the body, so you don't get dehydrated.

How to eat it
You can roast fennel with other vegetables or even boil, strain, and drink it as a tea.

Whether **cranberries** help prevent or treat UTI is still being debated, with recent studies suggesting they may not be able to lower the number of bacteria in women's urine. Still, the nutrients in these berries support immune-system health and may curb the risk of heart disease.

How to eat them
Cook cranberries and oranges or other citrus fruits on a stove top to make a jam.

Sage can be made into tea, is an ancient remedy for sore throats, cough, and colds. One Swiss study found that using sage with other herbs like echinacea can help relieve throat irritation.

How to eat it

Mix sage, goat cheese and eggs for a flavor-filled omelet. You can also add this earthy herb to bean soups and chicken, and beef dishes.

Garlic's scent tips you off to its many health benefits. The pungent aroma comes from sulfur compounds, including allicin. Scientists believe that allicin may block enzymes involved in infections; some studies suggest that swallowing garlic may ward off colds. (It can be easiest to eat garlic cooked with other foods, although some people can stomach eating a bit like a pill, followed by milk or water). Research has also linked garlic intake to a lower risk of stomach, colon, and esophagus cancers.

How to eat it

For a flavor and immunity boost, add garlic to marinades, roasted vegetables, or grain bowls.

Lemons are high in compounds called bioflavonoids, which kill cancer-causing free radicals. They also provide vitamin C (you can meet half your daily requirement from one fruit), so adding lemon juice to your meals is an easy strategy for protecting yourself against colds and other infections.

How to eat them

One simple way to work with a daily dose of vitamin C is to drink lemon water, either chilled or warm. A squeeze of lemon also makes steamed veggies tastier.

People who eat an **apple** a day use fewer prescription medications. And regular apple eaters report fewer asthma symptoms (a flavonoid called khellin may open airways). Apples are also high in fiber, which can help reduce the inflammation common during infections. Bonus: they're a superfood when it comes to satiety.

How to eat them

To turn apples into a more energizing snack, slice one up and enjoy with a spoonful of peanut or almond butter. Buy organic or wash well before eating: a recent study found that a little water and baking soda remove pesticide residue from the fruit.

Half a **grapefruit** has more than 60% of your daily vitamin C content, and eating grapefruit may also help the body absorb other essential nutrients, such as iron. People who regularly consume foods containing vitamin C may have slightly shorter colds or milder symptoms.

How to eat it
For a healthy morning treat, broiled grapefruit with a little cinnamon sugar.

Jalapeno peppers get their spice from a compound called capsaicin, which is something of an all-star in the nutrition world. Capsaicin acts as an anti-inflammatory agent and may ease arthritis symptoms. Some research suggests it can also keep your metabolism humming.

How to eat it
Add diced jalapeno peppers to guacamole for an extra kick of flavor. You can also mix these peppers into your favorite cornbread recipe.

One cup of alfalfa sprouts has less than 10 calories, is virtually fat-free, and contains phytochemicals called saponins, which may protect against cancer and help lower cholesterol. Enjoy their fresh, earthy crunch in salads or sandwiches or atop a lean turkey or veggie burger.

Apples are the richest fruit source of pectin, a soluble fiber that has been shown to lower blood pressure, reduce cholesterol, decrease the risk of colon and breast cancers, and even lessen the severity of diabetes.

Try throwing a few slices on your favorite sandwich or toss with field greens, toasted pecans, and a light vinaigrette for a delicious salad. With so many varieties available, you'll never get bored finding new ways to incorporate them into your daily diet.

Just one-half of a medium avocado contains more than 4 grams of fiber and 15% more than your recommended daily folate intake. Cholesterol-free and rich in monosaturated fats and potassium, avocados are powerful to the health of your heart. It also keeps you slim.

Use avocados as the base for a creamy homemade sandwich spread or add a few chunks to your favorite salsa for a simple and delicious way to dress up grilled chicken or fish.

Beets are loaded with antioxidants and have been found to protect against cancer, heart disease, and inflammation. Naturally sweet and full of fiber and vitamin C, beets make a delicious and nutrient-packed addition to any meal. Try finely grated raw beets in your salads or roast them along with sweet potatoes and parsnips for a colorful and flavorful side-dish—just keep in mind that certain cooking methods (like boiling) may decrease their nutritional value. And don't forget about the leafy green tops, which are rich in iron and folate, and can be prepared much like their cousins, Swiss chard and spinach.

Cranberries are renowned for protecting against urinary tract infections, but did you also know they may improve blood cholesterol and aid in recovery from strokes? Cranberry juice has also been shown to make cancer drugs more potent. Although available frozen year-round, enjoy these tart and tangy berries fresh during their peak season from farmer markets or grow them yourselves.

Not only does flaxseed lower blood cholesterol and reduce the risk of heart attack, it is also a rich source of lignan, a powerful antioxidant that may be a powerful ally against disease and certain cancers, especially breast cancer. Just 2 tablespoons of ground seeds (which are digested more efficiently than whole seeds) contain about 20% of the recommended daily fiber intake and more than 100% of the recommended intake for inflammation-fighting omega-3 fatty acids. Add ground flaxseed to baked goods for a nutty flavor, or sprinkle it on top of your favorite cereal. It's also delicious when blended with yogurt and fresh fruit for a tasty smoothie.

*One word of caution: Incorporate flaxseed into your diet gradually as it can have a laxative effect.

Just one medium orange (think tennis ball) supplies all your daily vitamin C, which is a dynamite immunity booster and cancer fighter. And consuming vitamin C is best done in its natural form. Italian researchers also found that test subjects had greater antioxidant protection after drinking orange juice versus vitamin C–fortified water. Plus, this sweet and tangy fruit is a good source of fiber, potassium, calcium, folate, and other B vitamins. The tangy taste of oranges makes a great combination with other strong flavors, such as ginger and honey. Put them on salads or use them in marinades and sauces for meats.

Trying to get more vitamin C in your diet? One cup of papaya cubes supplies more than 100% of your daily requirement, as well as a hefty dose of potassium and folate. It is also a good source of vitamins A and E, two powerful antioxidants that protect against heart disease and colon cancer. Savor the rich, buttery flesh of this tropical fruit in smoothies and salads, or simply scoop it out of the shell with a spoon.

This hearty, fiber-rich squash is packed with beta-carotene (converted to vitamin A in the body), which reduces the risk of developing lung cancer. The antioxidant activity of this vitamin combined with potassium, which may help prevent high blood pressure, makes it a nutritional superstar. If you prepare a whole squash, toast the seeds for a delicious snack containing heart-healthy fats. The sweet taste and moist texture make it ideal for desserts.

Packed with a variety of nutrients, including iron and copper, it's no wonder the Incas deemed this ancient seed "the mother of all grains." Quinoa contains all the essential amino acids, making it a complete protein (perfect for vegans and vegetarians). It is also a great source of magnesium, which relaxes blood vessels and has been found to reduce the frequency of migraines. Researchers have found that consuming dietary fiber, specifically from whole-grain products such as quinoa, reduces the risk of high blood pressure and heart attack.

Keep your heart in shape by substituting quinoa for rice or pasta in your next meal. Excellent base for seafood dishes and mixes well with beans.

Tart, sweet, and incredibly juicy, just one-half cup of these berries provides a whopping 4 grams of fiber and more than 25% of the daily recommended intake for both vitamin C and manganese. Raspberries also contain a powerful arsenal of antioxidants, including members of the anthocyanin family, which give raspberries their ruby-red hue and antimicrobial properties.

Try a few berries with your morning cereal or use them to add flavor to a green salad. Be adventurous and try with Arugula.

Powerful antioxidants in spinach have been found to combat a variety of cancers, including ovarian, breast, and colon cancers. And it's good for the noggin: Research indicates that spinach reduces the decline in brain function associated with aging and protects the heart from cardiovascular disease. Although it contains relatively high amounts of iron and calcium, oxalate compounds bind to these minerals and diminish their absorption.

Spinach has a mild flavor, so spice it up with garlic, olive oil, and onions.

Need a beta-carotene fix? Just one medium sweet potato packs over four times the recommended daily amount. These tasty tubers are also rich in potassium, inflammation-fighting vitamin C, and vitamin B6, which may prevent clogged arteries.

Boiling sweet potatoes may cause some of the water-soluble vitamins to leach out, so try them baked, roasted, or cubed, and added to soups or stews. If you need a boost of fiber, make sure to leave the skins on.

A 4-ounce portion of turkey breast meat contains 50% of your daily selenium, a trace mineral that plays essential roles in immune function and antioxidant defense. Despite the claim that turkey meat causes drowsiness during the holidays, it contains high amounts of niacin and vitamin B6, which are important for efficient energy production and blood-sugar regulation.

If you roast a whole bird, make sure to remove any skin, which is full of saturated fat; try substituting ground all-white-meat turkey breast for ground beef in your favorite hamburger recipe.

One-quarter cup of walnuts supplies 90% of the daily recommended amount of omega-3 fatty acids, which aid in everything from maintaining cognitive function to improving cholesterol and blood pressure.

Toss a few toasted walnut halves on your oatmeal (another heart-healthy superfood) or try them on your favorite salad for a tasty crunch.

Just 1 cup of watercress supplies 100% of a woman's recommended daily amount of vitamin K, which has been shown to prevent hardening of the arteries and is essential for strong bones. It is also a good source of vitamin A, a potent antioxidant. Try these peppery leaves in place of lettuce in salads or sandwiches or toss them in a quick stir-fry or soup.

Yogurt contains probiotics, which are bacteria that live in the intestine. It aid in digestion, boost the immune system, diminish bad breath, and are even associated with longer life spans. A 1-cup serving also supplies one-third of your daily calcium requirement, as well as 14 grams of satisfying protein. Opt for low-fat or nonfat versions to minimize saturated fat and try substituting plain yogurt for a healthier alternative to sour cream. Lactose intolerant? Look for soy or rice milk varieties.

Cooking Easy meal

Mushrooms stuffed with Crab

20 Cremini Mushrooms

10 ounces of crab meat finely chopped

½ cup softened cream cheese

4 cloves minced garlic

1tsp oregano

1tsbp chopped parsley

2tbsp grated Parmesan cheese

1. Preheat oven to 400 degrees placed parchment paper on a baking sheet.
2. Discard stems from the mushrooms. Clean each mushroom with a damp paper towel and place it on a baking sheet and sprinkle with sea salt.
3. Combine crab, cream cheese, garlic, oregano, and parsley in a mixing bowl and mix well.
4. Place the crab mixture in each mushroom cap. Sprinkle Parmesan cheese on the top of the stuffed mushrooms.

5. Bake the mushrooms until tender or 20-25 minutes as the crab stuffing is brown on top. Great appetizer or snack with honey lemon tea.

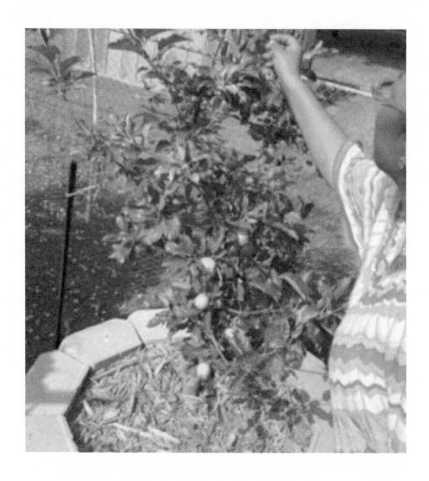

Time to Reflect on How This Changed Your Life

Will this motivate you to make positive changes? If so, how? (write your plans and the steps you will take to make changes)

_____

_____

_____

_____

_____

_____

_____

_____

_____

_____

_____

_____

_____

_____

_____

_____

_____

_____

_____

_____

_____

_____

_____

How did the chapter affect you and share your thoughts on how this information affects your life?

_____

_____

_____

_____

_____

_____

_____

_____

_____

_____

_____

_____

_____

_____

_____

_____

_____

_____

_____

_____

_____

_____

_____

_____

_____

_____

_____

_____

Where do you see yourself in a month or year after you consistently make these changes?

_____

_____

_____

_____

_____

_____

_____

_____

_____

_____

_____

_____

_____

_____

_____

_____

_____

_____

_____

_____

_____

_____

_____

Chapter Thirteen

BEAT BREAST CANCER. THE BATTLE IS WON

BREAST CANCER IS the most diagnosed cancer in women, and one in eight U.S. women will be diagnosed in her lifetime. The good news is that its incidence rates among women older than 50 have been on a slow decline, related to the decline in prescriptive hormone replacement therapy after menopause, which can increase breast cancer risk. What's more, death rates from breast cancer have been on the decline since the 1990s due to a combination of better screening, early detection, and improved treatment options. Although genetics play a role in our risk of breast cancer, lifestyle factors may also increase risk. These include a lack of physical activity, being overweight or obese, alcohol consumption, and eating a poor diet lacking in fruits and vegetables. When it comes to the last one, consider the foods that follow among your best dietary allies to help reduce your risk.

Blackberries: Increasing fiber intake is a smart strategy to help guard against breast cancer, and blackberries serve up 8 grams a cup. A 2016 study revealed that women who consumed the most fiber (versus the least) as teens and young adults had a significantly lower future risk of developing breast cancer. Plant fiber was especially beneficial.

A high-fiber diet helps lower circulating levels of estrogen; extended exposure to estrogen is thought to increase breast cancer risk. Fiber also helps control blood sugar, insulin, and insulin-like growth factors, which may be implicated in breast cancer.

♥ Also eat: Raspberries, kiwifruit, green peas, beans and lentils, sweet potato, bran cereals, whole grains.

Edamame: These fresh green soybeans are packed with isoflavones, phytochemicals linked with a lower risk of breast cancer recurrence and improved survival after breast cancer.

Studies conducted in breast cancer patients and survivors suggest that soy's protective effect is most apparent for women with aggressive forms of breast cancer that can't be treated with hormones. Found in grocery store freezers, edamame also delivers plant protein, fiber, and a decent amount of calcium, magnesium, and potassium.

Add shelled edamame to a stir-fry or soup near the end of cooking. Toss them into salads or grain bowls. Or steam or boil edamame in their pods and enjoy as a snack.

• Also eat soy flour, soy nuts, soy milk, tempeh, tofu.

*Disclaimer: I will not recommend these ingredients for men. It may lower the testosterone level.

Broccoli: Growing evidence suggests that eating vegetable guards against breast cancer, especially aggressive hormone-receptor negative breast cancers.

It's possible that antioxidants such as vitamins C and E, folate, phytochemicals, and fiber in vegetables have a synergistic effect when it comes to protection against breast cancer.

While all types of vegetables are beneficial, cruciferous veggies, such as broccoli, also supply anti-cancer isothiocyanates, phytochemicals that fend off harmful free radicals, quell inflammation and help the liver eliminate carcinogens. Add chopped broccoli to stir-fries, omelets, and frittatas. Top a baked potato or pizza with broccoli florets. Or serve it roasted or steamed as a side dish. The entire family will benefit from this meal.

Easy Meals

Broccoli Salad with Cucumber, avocado, and a boiled egg

2 cups of cucumber, sliced and seeded

4 cups of broccoli florets

2 boiled eggs chopped

1 large avocado diced

1/3 cup lemon juice

4 tsp olive oil

½ tsp honey

3 tsp Dijon mustard

Salt and pepper

1. Boil the broccoli florets in water for 6 minutes and rinse in cold water to stop the cooking process.
2. Add the broccoli to a large salad bowl with the chopped eggs, diced avocado, and sliced cucumbers.
3. Mix the mustard honey, olive oil, and lemon juice in a small mixing bowl and season with salt and pepper.
4. Pour the dressing over your salad and mix well. Enjoy healthy lunch, light dinner, or late snack.

Time to Reflect on How This Changed Your Life

Will this motivate you to make positive changes? If so, how? (write your plans and the steps you will take to make changes)

_____

_____

_____

_____

_____

_____

_____

_____

_____

_____

_____

_____

_____

_____

_____

_____

_____

_____

_____

_____

_____

_____

How did the chapter affect you and share your thoughts
on how this information affects your life?

_____

_____

_____

_____

_____

_____

_____

_____

_____

_____

_____

_____

_____

_____

_____

_____

_____

_____

_____

_____

_____

_____

_____

_____

_____

_____

_____

Where do you see yourself in a month or year after you consistently make these changes?

_____

_____

_____

_____

_____

_____

_____

_____

_____

_____

_____

_____

_____

_____

_____

_____

_____

_____

_____

_____

_____

_____

_____

_____

_____

Chapter Fourteen

WORD WORKS - SCRIPTURES

I. <u>Your health</u>

1 Corinthians 6:19-20
Don't you know that your body is the temple of the Holy Spirit, who lives in you and was given to you by God? You do not belong to yourself, for God bought you with a high price. So you must honor God with your body.

Psalm 38:3
Because of your anger, my whole body is sick; my health is broken because of my sins.

Proverbs 3:7-8
Don't be impressed with your own wisdom. Instead, fear the LORD and turn your back on evil. Then you will gain renewed health and vitality.

Proverbs 10:27
Fear of the LORD lengthens one's life, but the years of the wicked are cut short.

Proverbs 15:30
A cheerful look brings joy to the heart; good news makes for good health.

II.   <u>Emotional healing</u>

1 Peter 5:10
And after you have suffered a little while, the God of all grace, who has called you to his eternal glory in Christ, will himself restore, confirm, strengthen, and establish you.

Psalm 34:17-20
When the righteous cry for help, the Lord hears and delivers them out of all their troubles. The Lord is near to the brokenhearted and saves the crushed in spirit. Many are the afflictions of the righteous, but the Lord delivers him out of them all. He keeps all his bones; not one of them is broken.

Psalm 147:3
He heals the brokenhearted and binds up their wounds.

John 14:27
Peace I leave with you; my peace I give to you. Not as the world gives do I give to you. Let not your hearts be troubled, neither let them be afraid.

Exodus 14:14
The Lord will fight for you, and you have only to be silent.

III.   Stress release

John 14:27
Peace I leave with you; my peace I give you. I do not give to you as the world gives. Do not let your hearts be troubled and do not be afraid.

Romans 16:20
The God of peace will soon crush Satan under your feet. The grace of our Lord Jesus be with you.

Proverbs 16:3
Commit to the LORD whatever you do, and He will establish your plans.

Luke 21:19
Stand firm, and you will win life.

IV.   Uplift Yourself and Others

Proverbs 12:18
Some people make cutting remarks, but the words of the wise bring healing.

Proverbs 15:1
A gentle answer turns away wrath, but harsh words stir up anger.

Ephesians 4:32
Instead, be kind to each other, tenderhearted, forgiving one another, just as God through Christ has forgiven you.

Ephesians 4:29
Don't use foul or abusive language. Let everything you say be good and helpful, so that your words will be an encouragement to those who hear them.

V. Peace

Daniel 10:19
And he said, 'O man greatly loved, fear not, peace be with you; be strong and of good courage.' And as he spoke to me, I was strengthened and said, 'Let my lord speak, for you have strengthened me.'

John 16:33
"I have said these things to you, that in me you may have peace. In the world you will have tribulation. But take heart; I have overcome the world."

VI. <u>Loving your spouse/relationships</u>

Galatians 6:9
So, don't get tired of doing what is good. Don't get discouraged and give up, for we will reap a harvest of blessing at the appropriate time.

John 13:34
So now I am giving you a new commandment: Love each other. Just as I have loved you, you should love each other.

Romans 12:9,10
Don't just pretend that you love others. Really love them. Hate what is wrong. Stand on the side of the good. Love each other with genuine affection and take delight in honoring each other.

VI.   <u>Control Conflict</u>

Proverbs 25:19
Putting confidence in an unreliable person is like chewing with a toothache or walking on a broken foot.

Proverbs 12:25
Worry weighs a person down; an encouraging word cheers a person up.

Proverbs 17:22
A cheerful heart is good medicine, but a broken spirit saps a person's strength.

Matthew 6:34
"So don't worry about tomorrow, for tomorrow will bring its own worries. Today's trouble is enough for today."

VII. <u>Patient Parents</u>

Proverbs 22:6
Teach your children to choose the right path, and when they are older, they will remain upon it.

Proverbs 13:24
If you refuse to discipline your children, it proves you don't love them; if you love your children, you will be prompt to discipline them. (Do not belittle them, speak harsh or cause bodily harm. This is not of GOD – LaTonya).

Deuteronomy 6:6-7
And you must commit yourselves wholeheartedly to these commands I am giving you today. Repeat them again and again to your children. Talk about them when you are at home and when you are away on a journey, when you are lying down and when you are getting up again.

Colossians 3:21
Fathers, don't aggravate your children. If you do, they will become discouraged and quit trying.

VIII.   <u>Flowing Finances</u>

Ecclesiastes 5:10
Those who love money will never have enough. How absurd to think that wealth brings true happiness!

Proverbs 3:9-10
Honor the LORD with your wealth and with the best part of everything your land produces. Then He will fill your barns with grain, and your vats will overflow with the finest wine.

Proverbs 13:11
Wealth from get-rich-quick schemes quickly disappears; wealth from hard work grows.

Hebrews 13:5
Stay away from the love of money; be satisfied with what you have. For God has said, "I will never fail you. I will never forsake you."

Time to Reflect on How This Changed Your Life

Will this motivate you to make positive changes? If so, how? (write your plans and the steps you will take to make changes)

_____
_____
_____
_____
_____
_____
_____
_____
_____
_____
_____
_____
_____
_____
_____
_____
_____
_____
_____
_____
_____
_____
_____
_____

How did the chapter affect you and share your thoughts on how this information affects your life?

_____

_____

_____

_____

_____

_____

_____

_____

_____

_____

_____

_____

_____

_____

_____

_____

_____

_____

_____

_____

_____

_____

_____

_____

_____

_____

_____

Where do you see yourself in a month or year after you consistently make these changes?

_____

_____

_____

_____

_____

_____

_____

_____

_____

_____

_____

_____

_____

_____

_____

_____

_____

_____

_____

_____

_____

_____

_____

_____

_____

_____

Chapter Fifteen

GET YOUR PRAYERS WORKING

Our GOD does not care how you pray, but the fact that you spend time with HIM in a genuine way means so much. I like the way my pastor in St. Louis shares this message by stating you do not have to use fancy words, change your voice, or speak perfect grammar to talk with the LORD. You can't impress HIM. These are simple ways to communicate with GOD.

1. Be humble
2. Be persistent
3. Be consistent
4. Be bold with your words
5. Be in faith for your request
6. Be compassionate to others
7. Be in praise
8. Be in HIS will
9. Be ready to receive
10. Be in an agreement
11. Be blessed in your spirit, body, and mind. All other things will be a bonus.

Is anyone among you suffering? Let him pray. Is anyone cheerful? Let him sing praise. Is anyone among you sick? Let him call for the elders of the church, and let them pray over him, anointing him with oil in the name of the Lord. And the prayer of faith will save the one who is sick, and the Lord will raise him up. And if he has committed sins, he will be forgiven.

Time to Reflect on How This Changed Your Life

Will this motivate you to make positive changes? If so, how? (write your plans and the steps you will take to make changes)

_____

_____

_____

_____

_____

_____

_____

_____

_____

_____

_____

_____

_____

_____

_____

_____

_____

_____

_____

_____

_____

_____

_____

_____

How did the chapter affect you and share your thoughts on how this information affects your life?

_____

_____

_____

_____

_____

_____

_____

_____

_____

_____

_____

_____

_____

_____

_____

_____

_____

_____

_____

_____

_____

_____

_____

_____

_____

_____

_____

_____

Where do you see yourself in a month or year after you
consistently make these changes?

_____

_____

_____

_____

_____

_____

_____

_____

_____

_____

_____

_____

_____

_____

_____

_____

_____

_____

_____

_____

_____

_____

_____

_____

_____

Acknowledgments

Thank you for allowing me to share my story and celebrate my victory of healing. We are here to support each other and make the world a better place. Take time to love yourself. Be grateful for what you have. Compliment others with a sincere tone, not expecting anything in return. Speak with kindness, yet firm. We must stand for righteousness, peace and live a full, healthy, happy life with security.

Invest in your community and support those who need growth.

References:

THE HOLY BIBLE (King James Version)

William Chey, MD

Dr. Fuhrman

Journal Neurology 2018

Journal of Cellular Physiology 2017